My Mediterranean Lunch & Dinner

50 Quick, Easy & Delicious Recipes for Your Daily Mediterranean Meals

Jenna Violet

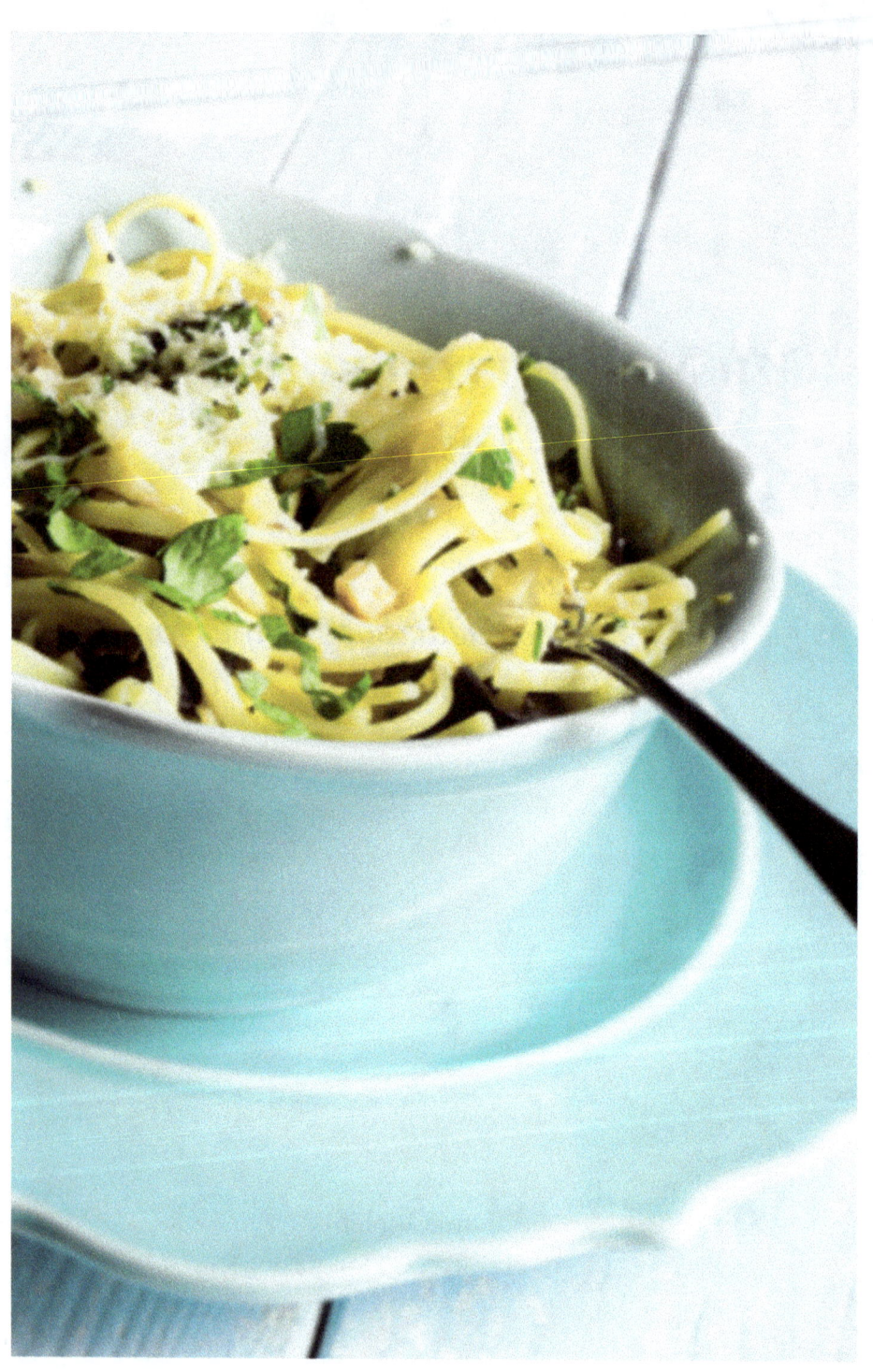

© Copyright 2021 - All rights reserved.

The content contained within this book may not be reproduced, duplicated or transmitted without direct written permission from the author or the publisher.
Under no circumstances will any blame or legal responsibility be held against the publisher, or author, for any damages, reparation, or monetary loss due to the information contained within this book. Either directly or indirectly.

Legal Notice:
This book is copyright protected. This book is only for personal use. You cannot amend, distribute, sell, use, quote or paraphrase any part, or the content within this book, without the consent of the author or publisher.

Disclaimer Notice:
Please note the information contained within this document is for educational and entertainment purposes only. All effort has been executed to present accurate, up to date, and reliable, complete information. No warranties of any kind are declared or implied. Readers acknowledge that the author is not engaging in the rendering of legal, financial, medical or professional advice. The content within this book has been derived from various sources. Please consult a licensed professional before attempting any techniques outlined in this book.

By reading this document, the reader agrees that under no circumstances is the author responsible for any losses, direct or indirect, which are incurred as a result of the use of information contained within this document, including, but not limited to, — errors, omissions, or inaccuracies.

Table of Contents

Roasted red pepper hummus 7

Roasted garlic hummus dip 9

Antipasto skewers 11

Baked rice recipe with jam and nuts 13

Lentil and rice with crispy onion 15

Vegan chili with quinoa 17

Easy ratatouille recipe 20

Easy butternut squash recipe with lentils and quinoa 24

Vegetarian egg casserole 27

Feta and spinach frittata 29

Simple roasted carrots recipe 32

Pesto pasta recipe with tomatoes and mozzarella 34

Vegetarian sweet potatoes stew 36

Eggplant recipe 38

Easy vegetarian pasta Faggioli recipe 40

Cinnamon roasted sweet potatoes 42

Greek stuffed tomatoes 44

Carpers chicken 47

Mediterranean potato hash with asparagus, chickpeas and poached eggs 49

Fried eggplant recipe with green peppers and tomatoes 51

Crunchy roasted chickpeas 53

Mediterranean style okra recipe 54

Mediterranean salmon and vegetable quinoa 56

Vegan tofu tikka masala 58

Mediterranean couscous 61

Stuffed peppers 63

Easy Falafel meal 65

Pan seared salmon 67

One pan baked cod and vegetables 70

Quinoa bowls with roasted pepper.. 71

Sweet potato wedges with tahini 73

Armenia losh kebab 75

Eggplant, lentils and pepper cooked in olive oil.. 77

Potato omelet 79

Eggs poached in spicy tomato sauce, the Moroccan style 81

Briam baked vegetables in olive oil 83

Eggplant parmesan with prosciutto 84

Lebanese hummus 86

Grilled swordfish with lemon parsley topping 87

Orange lemon potatoes 88

Chickpea patties with sesame, cilantro and parsley 89

Shrimp with feta and tomatoes 91

Seared scallops with lemon orzo 92

Pasta with sundried tomato pesto and feta cheese 94

Linguine with garlicky clams and peas 96

Toum garlic sauce 98

Eggplant rollatini recipe 100

Vegetarian moussaka recipe 102

Honey mustard salmon recipe 106

Muhammara recipe/roasted red pepper dip 108

Roasted red pepper hummus

This is a perfect Mediterranean diet twist with a delicious red pepper roast. It features sumac, smoked paprika, garlic and jalapeno.

Ingredients
- 1 lemon, juice of 1 lemon
- 1 jalapeno pepper, sliced in half length wise
- Salt
- 2 cups of cooked chickpeas
- 2 tablespoons of toasted pine nuts
- 4 garlic cloves, chopped
- Extra virgin olive oil
- 1 red bell pepper, seeded
- 5 tablespoons of tahini paste
- 4g of sumac
- ½ teaspoon of to 1 tsp smoked paprika

Directions
- Preheat your oven to 450°F.
- Place the red bell pepper strips and jalapeno in a small baking dish.
- Drizzle generously with olive oil.
- Place in the preheated oven and bake for 20 minutes until tender.
- Remove and drain any excess oil.

- Add the roasted bell peppers and jalapeno together with the chickpeas, garlic, tahini, smoked paprika, sumac, and lemon juice in a large food processor bowl.
- Drizzle a little extra virgin olive oil.
- Run the processor until desired creamy paste consistency.
- Test and adjust accordingly.
- Run the processor again to combine.
- Transfer to a serving bowl. Cover and let chill in a fridge.
- Serve and enjoy topped with roasted red pepper hummus with a little more extra virgin olive oil with a pinch of paprika.

Roasted garlic hummus dip

It is a silky creamy dip very sweet and smoky with enough zing. Feel free to top with pine nuts and feta.

Ingredients

- ½ teaspoon of cayenne pepper
- [Private Reserve](#) Greek extra virgin olive oil
- 1 teaspoon of [za'atar spice](#)
- 2 ½ cup of cooked chickpeas
- Crumbled feta cheese
- 4 tablespoons of [tahini](#)
- Toasted pine nuts
- 3 tablespoons of fresh lemon juice
- 2 heads of garlic
- 2 tablespoons of water, more as needed
- Salt
- 1 teaspoon of [sumac](#)
- 3 tablespoons of chopped fresh parsley

Directions

- Preheat your oven to 400°F.
- Place the garlic cloves each in a piece of foil that's large enough to wrap around.
- Lightly drizzle with olive oil.
- Close the foil up.
- Bake in the preheated oven for 45 minutes or until the garlic is soft.

- Remove from heat and let cool briefly, then peel.
- In the bowl of a food processor, fitted with a blade, place the roasted garlic, chickpeas, lemon juice, tahini, and water.
- Sprinkle salt, sumac and cayenne.
- Then, blend until smooth, you can water if dry.
- Taste and adjust accordingly.
- Spread the roasted garlic hummus in a bowl.
- Add a generous drizzle of quality extra virgin olive oil.
- Top with za'atar spice or parsley, toasted pine nuts, and crumbled feta if desired.
- Serve with warm pita bread and enjoy.

Antipasto skewers

This recipe is another vegetable blast of a Mediterranean diet. It features marinated vegetables and herbs with festive appetizers to pull the crowd.

Ingredients
- 10 pitted Kalamata olives
- 10 mini wooden skewers
- Drizzle extra virgin olive oil
- 20 flat-leaf parsley
- 10 pieces of preserved artichoke hearts
- 10 cherry tomatoes
- 10 pieces of prosciutto di Parma
- Pinch of dried oregano
- 10 mini mozzarella cheese balls

Directions
- Soak mini wooden skewers in water for one hour.
- Make sure to Pat dry.
- Skewer the antipasto ingredients beginning perhaps with the basil or parsley, followed by the larger pieces like prosciutto or artichoke hearts.
- Place the Kalamata olive at the very top of the skewer.
- Arrange skewers on a serving platter.

- Sprinkle with dried oregano and drizzle of extra virgin olive oil.
- Serve cold or at room temperature.
- Enjoy.

Baked rice recipe with jam and nuts

Ingredients
- ⅓ cup of shelled pistachios roughly chopped
- 3 tablespoon of fig jam or honey divided
- 13 ounces of round French brie
- ¼ cup of dried mission figs sliced
- ¼ cup of walnut hearts roughly chopped

Directions
- Preheat the oven to 375°F.
- Place the fig jam in a microwave-safe dish.
- Microwave for 30 seconds to soften.
- In a small bowl, combine the sliced dried figs with the nuts.
- Add half of the fig jam and mix well to coat with the nut mixture.
- Place the round of brie in a small cast iron skillet.
- Using a knife, coat the brie with the remainder of the jam.
- Top the brie with the fig and nut mixture.
- Place the dish on top of a baking sheet.
- Bake on the middle rack of your heated oven for 15 minutes.
- Remove from the oven and let the brie settle for 5 minutes.

- Serve warm and enjoy with favorite crackers.

Lentil and rice with crispy onion

This recipe is flavored with the crispy onions, a strong signature copied to the Mediterranean diet from the eastern dishes. It is similar to the Lebanese rose water and orange blossoms.

Ingredients
- 1 cup of black lentils , sorted and rinsed
- Parsley or parsley flakes
- Black pepper
- Oil for frying
- 4 cups of water, divided
- ¼ cup of private reserve Greek extra virgin olive oil
- 2 large yellow onions, diced
- 1 large yellow onion cut in very thin rings
- 1 teaspoon of kosher salt
- 1 cup of long-grain white rice, soaked in water

Directions
- Place the lentils in a small saucepan with 2 cups of the water.
- Boil over high heat
- Lower the heat let simmer while cover until the lentils are par-boiled for 12 minutes.
- Remove from heat source, drain any excess water then set aside.

- In a large pan, heat oil over medium-high heat.
- Add the diced onions and cook until the onions are dark golden brown for 40 minutes.
- Sprinkle the onions with a teaspoon of salt as they cook.
- Add the remaining 2 cups of water.
- Boil over high heat, and then reduce the heat to low let simmer for 2 minutes.
- Stir the rice and par-cooked lentils into the onion mixture.
- Cover and bring back to a boil.
- Stir in a healthy pinch of salt and the black pepper.
- Reduce the heat to low, cover to absorb any excess liquid in 20 minutes.
- Remove from heat.
- Season with salt and pepper to taste.
- Serve the Mujadara hot or at room temperature with a drizzle of extra virgin olive oil and parsley garnish, if desired.
- Enjoy.

Vegan chili with quinoa

This is a huge Mediterranean bold twist with a protein power house featuring two different kind of beans with variety of chopped vegetables and packed with rich refreshing flavors.

Ingredients
- ½ teaspoon of ground allspice
- 1 cup of water
- 1 large lime juice of
- ½ large yellow onion chopped
- 1 teaspoon of ground cumin
- ¼ cup of chopped fresh parsley
- 5 garlic cloves minced
- 2 carrots peeled and chopped
- ½ cup of quinoa uncooked
- ½ large green bell pepper chopped
- 1 16-ounces of chopped tomatoes with juice
- 4 cups of low-sodium vegetable broth
- Greek extra virgin olive oil
- 2 ½ teaspoon of chili powder
- 1 15- ounces of kidney beans drained and rinsed
- 1 teaspoon of sweet paprika
- Salt and pepper
- 1 15- ounces of black beans drained and rinsed

- ½ cup of chopped fresh cilantro
- 1 jalapeno sliced

Directions
- In a small saucepan, combine quinoa and water.
- Cook over medium heat for 15 minutes until the water is absorbed.
- Remove from heat and set aside for later.
- In large saucepan, heat 2 tablespoon of extra virgin olive oil over medium heat until shimmering without smoke.
- Add onions, garlic, carrots, and bell peppers.
- Cook for 4 minutes, tossing regularly to softened.
- Add tomatoes, broth, and spices.
- Season with salt and pepper.
- Bring to a boil.
- Stir in black beans, kidney beans, and partially-cooked quinoa.
- Reduce the heat let simmer for 25 minutes.
- Remove from heat source.
- Stir in cilantro, parsley, and lemon juice.
- Transfer to serving bowls, drizzle with early harvest extra virgin olive oil and jalapeno slices.
- Serve and enjoy.

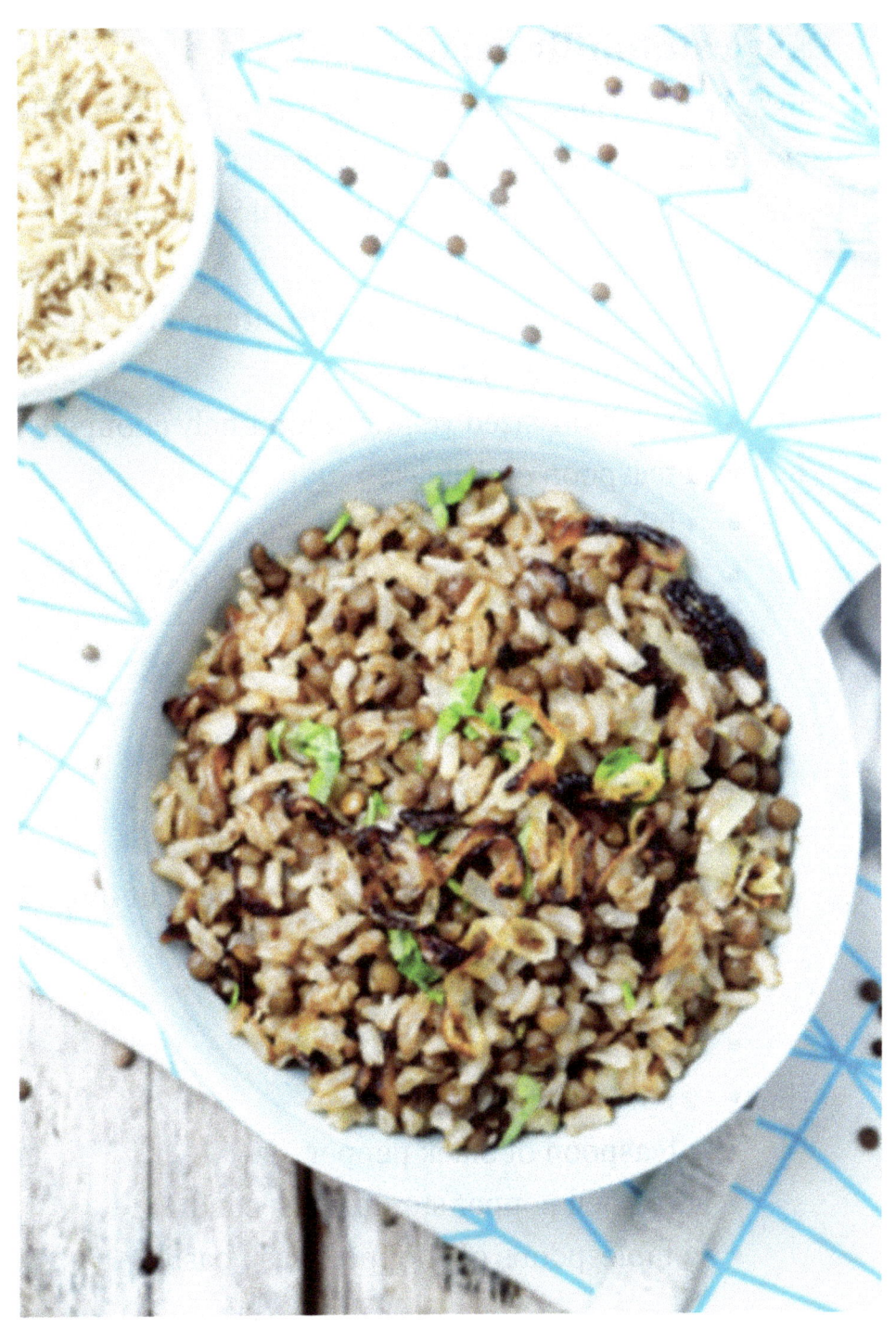

Easy ratatouille recipe

This a typical classic Mediterranean Sea diet vegetable stew features several vegetables especially eggplants, tomatoes, summer squash, flavorful garlic and onions.

Ingredients

- [Private reserve]() Greek extra virgin olive oil
- Eggs over-easy fried
- 1 medium-sized yellow onion finely chopped
- 1 teaspoon of [dried rosemary]()
- 1 tablespoon of sherry vinegar
- 1 green bell pepper stemmed, seeded
- Crusty bread
- 1 lb. eggplant peeled
- 6 garlic cloves peeled, and minced
- 1 teaspoon of [sweet paprika]()
- 2 lb. of vine ripe tomatoes chopped
- 2 zucchini halved length-wise, then cut into ½ inch pieces
- Kosher salt
- ½ cup of red wine
- 2 springs of fresh thyme
- 1 teaspoon of black pepper
- 1 red bell pepper stemmed, seeded
- 3 tablespoons of chopped fresh basil

Directions

- Place eggplant pieces in a large colander over your sink.
- Sprinkle with salt let stay for 20 minutes as the eggplant sweats out its bitterness.
- Pat dry to remove water.
- In a large heavy pot, heat 2 tablespoons of extra virgin olive oil over medium heat until shimmering without smoke.
- Add the onions.
- Let cook while stirring regularly, until onions turn translucent.
- Now add the red peppers together with the green peppers, continue to cook for 4 minutes, stir.
- Add the garlic, zucchini, tomatoes, wine, eggplant, and fresh thyme springs.
- Stir in black pepper, paprika, and rosemary.
- Season with kosher salt and adjust accordingly.
- Raise the heat to medium-high, bring to a boil for 5 minutes, stirring twice.
- Turn down the heat, then cover and cook over low heat for 20 minutes.
- Remove the ratatouille from the heat.
- Taste and adjust seasoning accordingly.

- Add the sherry vinegar and drizzle with extra virgin olive oil.
- Top with fresh basil.
- Transfer the ratatouille to dinner bowls, top each with a fried egg and add crusty bread on the side.
- Serve and enjoy.

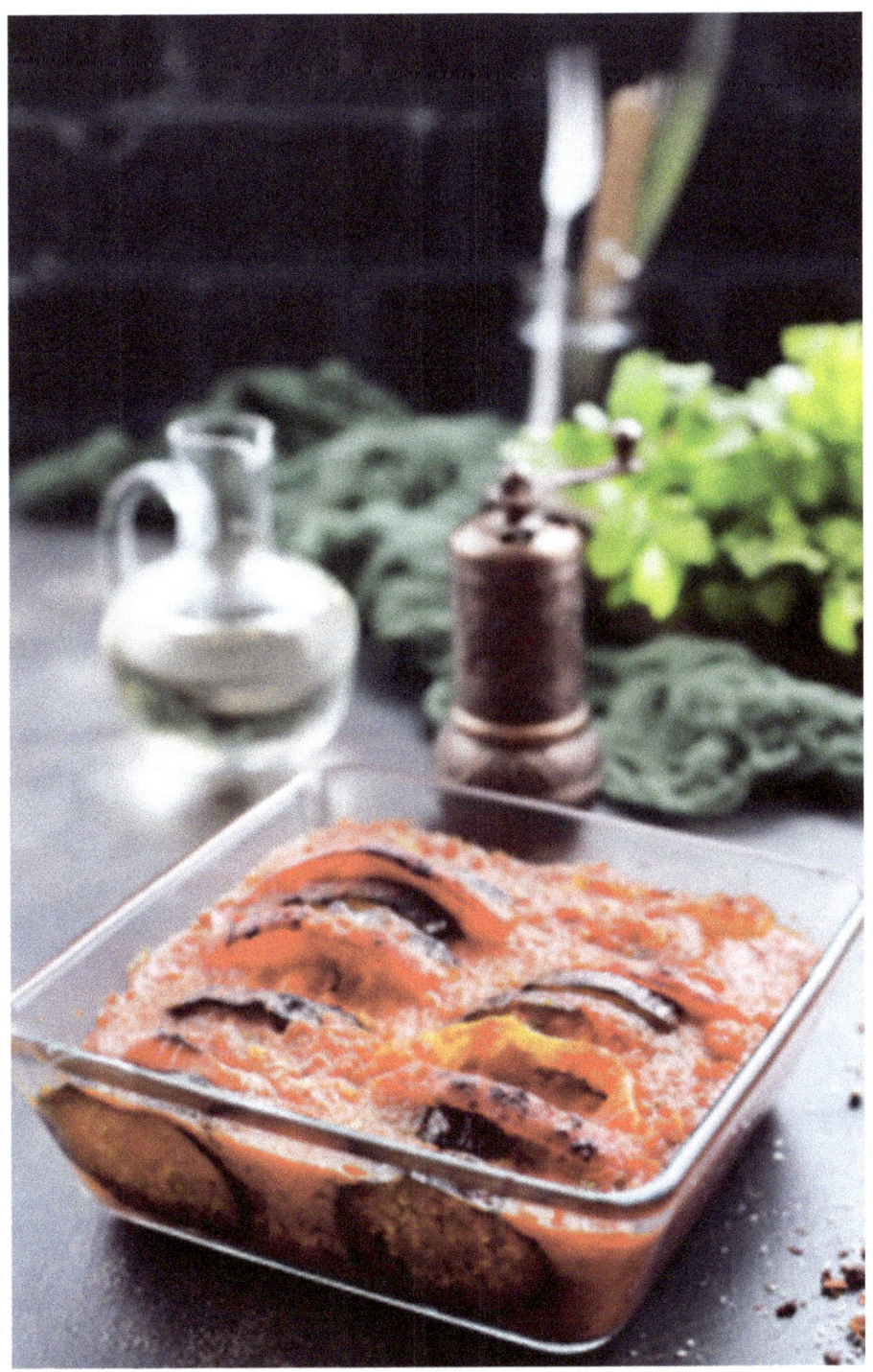

Easy butternut squash recipe with lentils and quinoa

This recipe is augmented with lentils and quinoa for a satisfying lunch with Mediterranean diet spices an extra crunch derived from roasted almonds and warm fall salad.

Ingredients

- Large handful of fresh parsley, chopped
- 1 whole butternut squash
- Salt
- 2 teaspoons of allspice , divided
- ½ cup of toasted slivered almonds
- Fresh lemon juice
- 1 teaspoon of coriander , divided
- 1 teaspoon of paprika , divided
- 6 garlic cloves, peeled
- Private reserve extra virgin olive oil
- 1 cup of dry quinoa
- 1 cup of dry black lentils, sorted and rinsed
- Water
- 2 scallions, white and green parts, trimmed and chopped
- ¾ teaspoon of cumin
- 2 teaspoons of ground cinnamon, divided

Directions

- Preheat oven to 425°F.

- Microwave butternut squash for 3 minutes.
- Place cubed butternut squash on a large baking sheet.
- Season with salt.
- Sprinkle with cinnamon, allspice, coriander, paprika, and cumin.
- Drizzle with private reserve extra virgin olive oil and toss.
- Spread the squash in one layer on the sheet pan.
- Place on the middle rack of heated oven.
- When ready fried in 15 minutes, remove and add the garlic cloves and drizzle with a little olive oil. Toss squash cubes.
- Return to oven for another 10 minutes.
- Place black lentils in a sauce pan and add 3 cups of water.
- Season with salt boil.
- Lower the heat let simmer for 25 minutes.
- Drain any excess oil.
- Place rinsed quinoa in another saucepan.
- Add 2 cups of water.
- Season with salt, boil, then lower heat let simmer for 20 minutes.
- Place cooked lentils and quinoa in a large bowl.

- Season with the remainder of spices and a little salt.
- Toss a little to combine.
- Add the cooked butternut squash.
- Chop the roasted garlic and add together with the scallions and fresh parsley.
- Toss all the ingredients together.
- Add fresh lemon juice to your taste
- Add a generous drizzle of extra virgin olive oil. Toss.
- Taste and adjust accordingly and top with tomatoes.
- Serve warm and enjoy.

Vegetarian egg casserole

This is a non-static Mediterranean vegetable recipe. It is versatile, in that you change the veggies according to your liking.

Ingredients

- 4 ounces of artichoke hearts
- 3 ounces of crumbled feta cheese
- 1 ounce of chopped fresh parsley
- ½ teaspoon of baking powder
- Kosher salt and black pepper
- 3 ounces of sliced mushrooms
- 1 bell pepper sliced into rounds
- 1 teaspoon of dry oregano
- 8 large eggs
- 1 teaspoon of [sweet paprika](#)
- Extra virgin olive oil
- ¼ teaspoon of [nutmeg](#)
- 1 ½ cups of milk
- 3 slices bread cut into ½ inch pieces
- 2 shallots, thinly sliced
- 1 tomato, small diced
- 2 ounces of pitted Kalamata olives, sliced

Directions

- Start by heating your oven to 375°F.

- In a large mixing bowl, whisk together the eggs, milk, baking powder, salt, pepper, and spices.
- Add the bread pieces, artichoke hearts, shallots, mushrooms, tomatoes, Kalamata olives, feta and parsley. Mix.
- Lightly brush the casserole dish with extra virgin olive oil.
- Transfer the egg and vegetable mixture into the casserole dish and spread evenly.
- Organize the bell pepper slices on top.
- Bake for about 35 to 45 minutes.
- Let the casserole to settle.
- Cut through and serve.
- Enjoy.

Feta and spinach frittata

Ingredients

- 1 teaspoon of dried oregano
- Extra virgin olive oil
- ½ teaspoon of dill weed
- 3 tablespoons of chopped fresh mint leaves
- 3 garlic cloves, minced
- ½ teaspoon of black pepper
- ¼ cup of milk
- 4 ounces of crumbled feta cheese
- 8 eggs
- ½ teaspoon of paprika
- ¼ teaspoon of baking powder
- pinch salt
- 6 ounces of frozen chopped spinach
- ½ cup finely chopped yellow onion
- 1 cup chopped fresh parsley

Directions

- Preheat your oven to 375°F.
- In a large bowl, whisk together eggs, spices, baking powder, and pinch of salt.
- Add spinach and all remaining ingredients to the egg mixture. Mix.
- In a skillet, heat 2 tablespoons of olive oil until shimmering without smoke.

- Pour in the egg mixture. shake to allow the egg mixture to spread well.
- Cook on medium-high heat for 4 minutes.
- Transfer to heated oven to finish cooking for 8 minutes.
- Serve and enjoy with 3 ingredient Mediterranean salad.

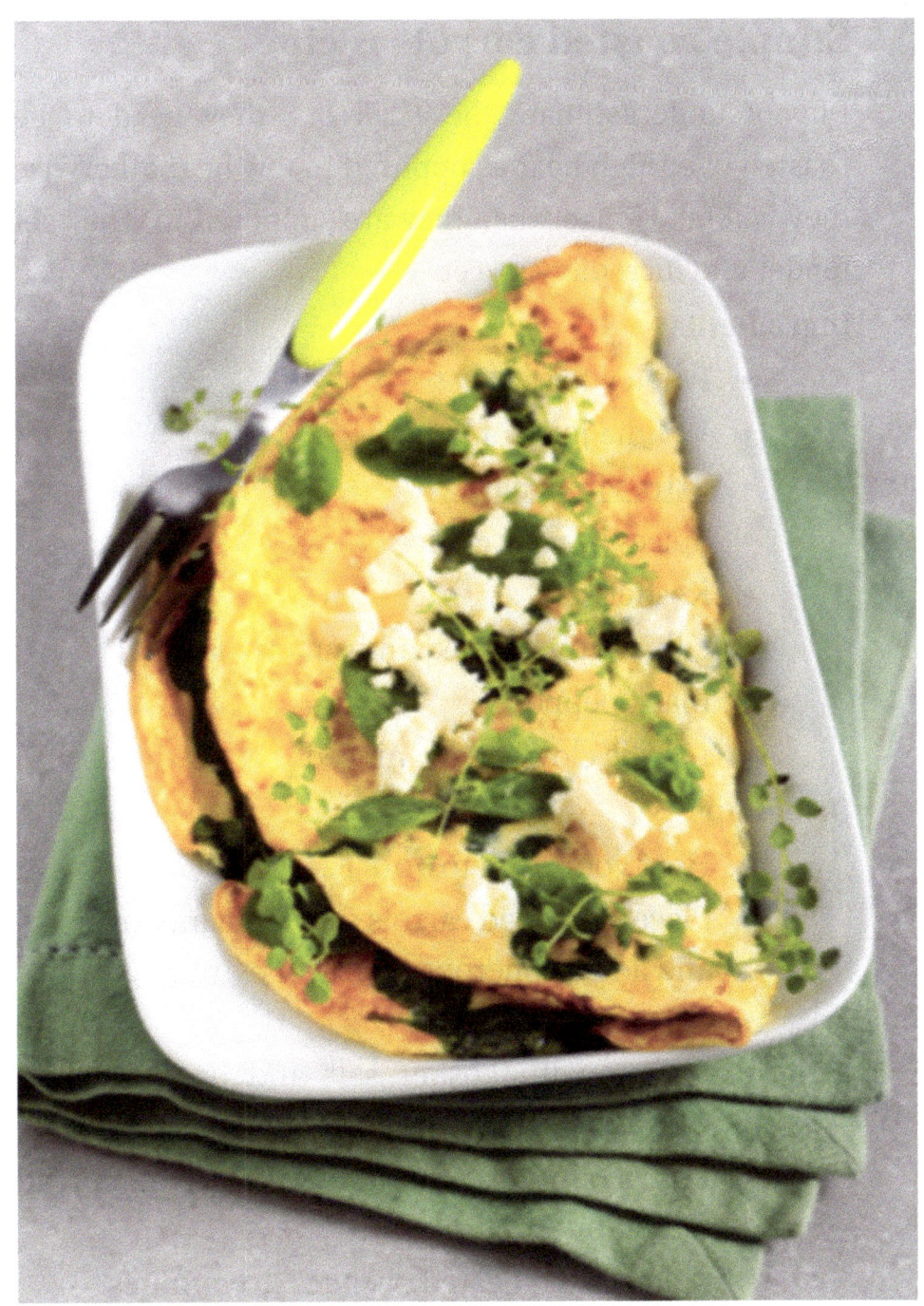

Simple roasted carrots recipe

Do not underestimate these carrots, they need to be roasted over high heat as opposed to low heat otherwise they will take longer than they are supposed to. They get tender and incredibly sweet.

Ingredients
- Parsley for garnish
- ½ lime juice of lemon
- [Extra virgin olive oil](#)
- Spices of your choice
- Kosher salt
- 2 lb. carrots peeled and cut on diagonal
- Black pepper
- 1 garlic clove finely minced

Directions
- Heat your oven to 400°F.
- Place the sliced carrots in a large mixing bowl, and add a generous drizzle of extra virgin olive oil.
- Season with kosher salt and black pepper. Toss.
- Transfer the carrots to a baking pan, spread well in one single layer.
- Roast in the heated oven for 30 minutes.

- Turn carrots over to get even color on both sides.
- Transfer the roasted carrots to a serving bowl.
- Add flavor to your liking.
- Season with turmeric and harissa spice blend.
- If desired, add a little minced garlic and a splash of lime juice.
- Serve and enjoy.

Pesto pasta recipe with tomatoes and mozzarella

The pesto pasta recipe is a perfect coat for the pasta with sauce to attain a maximum flavor with juicy roasted tomatoes and frozen mozzarella for a perfect Mediterranean diet dinner.

Ingredients
- 6 ounces of fresh baby mozzarella
- 1 cup of basil pesto
- 2 lb.. small tomatoes halved
- Fresh basil for garnish
- Kosher salt and black pepper
- [Extra virgin olive oil](#)
- 1 lb.. thin spaghetti
- 2 garlic cloves minced

Directions
- Start by heating your oven to 450°F.
- In a larger bowl, toss the tomatoes with kosher salt, black pepper, garlic and extra virgin olive oil.
- Transfer to a sheet-pan and bake in heated oven for 35 minutes.
- As the tomatoes roast, cook the spaghetti in boiling water as per the package Directions.

- Drain any excess water, reserving ½ cup for later.
- Transfer the cooked spaghetti to a large bowl.
- Add the pesto and toss to coat.
- Taste and adjust the seasoning accordingly.
- Add the roasted tomatoes and mozzarella to the bowl of pasta, toss.
- Serve and enjoy warm with basil if you desire.

Vegetarian sweet potatoes stew

This is a whole meal fit for breakfast, lunch, and dinner. It is loaded with potatoes with a natural Mediterranean Sea diet sweetness elevated by tomatoes, carrots and silted baby spinach.

Ingredients
- 5 ounces of baby spinach
- 1 teaspoon of ground coriander
- Extra virgin olive oil
- 1 large yellow onion, chopped
- 4 garlic cloves, minced
- 3 carrots, peeled and chopped
- 1 cup of chopped fresh parsley
- 3 sweet potatoes, peeled and cubed
- ¾ teaspoon of Aleppo pepper
- Kosher salt and pepper
- ½ teaspoon of turmeric
- 1 15 ounces of can diced tomatoes with their juices
- 1 teaspoon of ground cumin
- 3 cups low-sodium vegetable broth

Directions
- In a small bowl, add coriander, Aleppo pepper, cumin, and turmeric. Mix, set aside.

- In a large heavy pot, heat 2 tablespoon of extra virgin olive oil over medium heat until shimmering.
- Add onions and garlic let cook for 3 minutes, stirring occasionally.
- Add carrots together with sweet potatoes.
- Season with kosher salt, black pepper, and the spice mixture.
- Increase the heat to high, let cook for 5 minutes, stirring occasionally.
- Add diced tomatoes and broth, boil for 10 minutes.
- Lower the heat, cover halfway and let simmer 25 minutes.
- Stir in the baby spinach and fresh parsley.
- Remove from heat, drizzle with extra virgin olive oil.
- Serve and enjoy with crusty bread.

Eggplant recipe

These eggplants are perfected to velvet tender wit chickpeas and tomatoes. It is richly vegan with great garlic and onion flavors.

Ingredients

- 1 teaspoon of dry oregano
- 1.5 lb. eggplant, cut into cubes
- ½ teaspoon of organic ground turmeric
- 1 28-ounces of can chopped tomato
- ¾ teaspoon of ground cinnamon
- Fresh herbs
- Kosher salt
- Extra virgin olive oil
- 1 large yellow onion, chopped
- ½ teaspoon of black pepper
- 1 teaspoon of organic ground coriander
- 1 green bell pepper, stem and innards removed, diced
- 2 15-ounces of cans chickpeas
- 1 carrot, chopped
- 6 large garlic cloves, minced
- 2 dry bay leaves
- 1 ½ teaspoons of sweet paprika

Directions

- Heat your oven to 400°F.

- Place eggplant cubes in a colander over a large bowl and sprinkle with salt.
- Set aside for 20 minutes to sweat out any bitterness.
- Rinse with water and pat dry.
- In a large saucepan, heat extra virgin olive oil over medium-high until shimmering without smoke.
- Add onions together with the peppers, and chopped carrot.
- Let cook for 3 minutes, stirring regularly.
- Add garlic together with the bay leaf, spices, and a dash of salt.
- Continue to cook 1 minute, stirring until fragrant.
- Add eggplant with the chickpeas, chopped tomato, and reserved chickpea liquid. Stir.
- Bring to a rolling boil for 10 minutes, stir often.
- Remove from stove top, cover and transfer to oven.
- Cook in oven for 45 minutes.
- Add a generous drizzle of extra virgin olive oil when the eggplants are ready, then garnish with fresh herbs.
- Serve and enjoy when warm.

Easy vegetarian pasta Faggioli recipe

This is a heaty and rusty Italian bowl with a Mediterranean twist especially roasted tomatoes, beans and some tender nutritious veggies.

Ingredients
- Extra virgin olive oil
- 6 cups of vegetable broth
- Grated Parmesan cheese
- 1 28-ounces of can fire roasted diced tomatoes
- 2 carrots, chopped
- Crushed red pepper
- 2 garlic cloves, chopped
- 1 dried bay leaf
- 1 teaspoon of dried oregano
- 1 yellow onion, chopped
- 8 ounces of small pasta
- 1 15-ounces of can cannellini beans
- 1 15-ounces of can kidney beans, rinsed and drained
- 2 celery stalks, chopped
- Salt and pepper
- ½ cup of fresh basil leaves, cut into ribbons

Directions
- In a large boiling pot of water, cook the pasta as per the manufacturers package Directions.

- Drain any excess water, and set aside.
- In a large cast iron pot, heat 2 tablespoon of olive oil.
- Sauté the onions, celery and carrots on medium-high heat for 4 minutes.
- Add the chopped garlic with the bay leaf and dried oregano.
- Cook for more 2 minutes, stirring occasionally.
- Add the roasted diced tomatoes with the vegetable broth, cannellini beans, and kidney beans.
- Season with salt and pepper.
- Boil, then reduce the heat to simmer.
- Cover the pot with a lid with a small opening. Simmer for 15 minutes.
- Bring to a medium-high heat.
- Stir in the pasta until warmed through.
- Stir in the fresh basil, and remove from heat.
- Transfer to serving bowls and top with crushed red pepper.
- Serve and enjoy with crusty bread.

Cinnamon roasted sweet potatoes

These potatoes are best roasted with red onions. The hint of cinnamon gives this recipe a deeper depth of flavor.

Ingredients
- 2 small red onions cut into large pieces
- 3 lb. sweet potatoes peeled and cut into cubes
- Black pepper
- 1 teaspoon of ground cinnamon
- Kosher salt
- Extra virgin olive oil
- ¾ teaspoon of ground allspice

Directions
- Begin by preheating your oven to 400°F.
- Place the sweet potato cubes together with the onion pieces in a large mixing bowl.
- Add a drizzle of extra virgin olive oil.
- Add salt, pepper, cinnamon and allspice. Toss.
- Shift to a sheet pan.
- Spread the sweet potatoes and onions well in one single layer without overcrowding.
- Roast for 45 minutes, tossing occasionally.
- Serve and enjoy when the potatoes are cooked through.

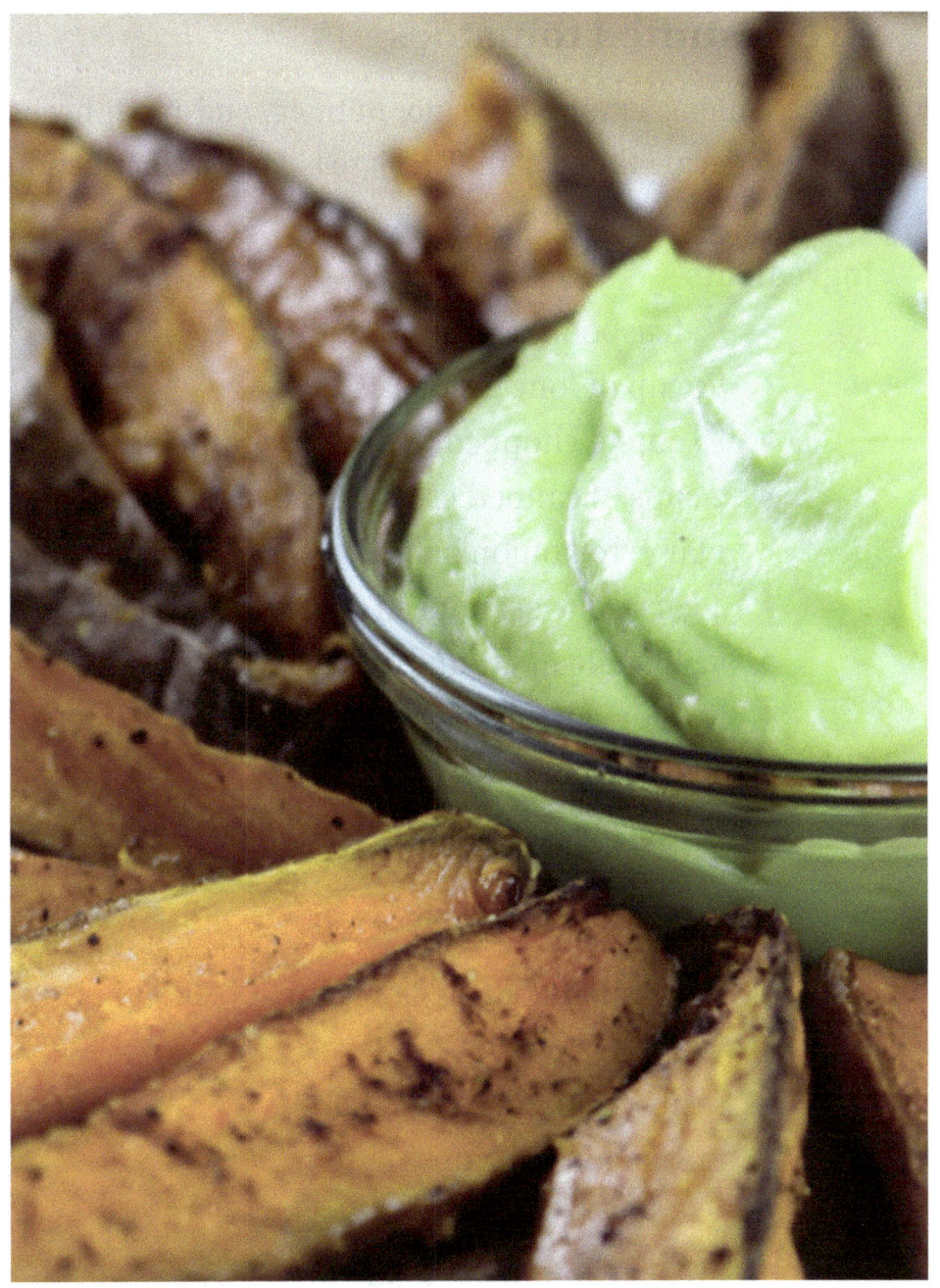

Greek stuffed tomatoes

Garlic, onions, cumin, oregano, nutmeg, and fresh herbs give this recipe thumbs up. They are baked to a perfection as they are stuffed with tomatoes.

Ingredients

- ½ teaspoon of ground nutmeg
- ½ cup of long grain rice
- ½ cup of chopped fresh spearmint
- 2 cups of canned crushed tomatoes
- 1 large red onion halved, mince ½ of the onion
- 4 garlic cloves, minced
- ½ lb. of lean ground beef
- Kosher salt and black pepper
- 6 large tomatoes
- ½ teaspoon of allspice
- ½ cup of white wine
- Extra virgin olive oil
- ¾ teaspoon of dried oregano
- ¼ cup of water
- 1 cup of chopped fresh parsley
- 1 teaspoon of ground cumin

Directions

- Preheat your oven ready to 375°F.
- Place olive oil in a large skillet over medium-high heat let shimmer without smoke.

- Add chopped onions and garlic, toss.
- Add the ground meat, season with salt, pepper, cumin, oregano, allspice, and nutmeg. Let cook for 5 minutes.
- Add drained rice when the meat is ready.
- Add crushed tomatoes, white wine, and water.
- Bring the saucy mixture to a boil, turn the heat down, let simmer for 10 minutes.
- Stir in the fresh herbs. Season with kosher salt.
- Oil the bottom of a baking pan with extra virgin olive oil.
- Spread chopped tomato flesh and sliced onion at the bottom of the baking dish.
- Add the chopped tomato flesh and sliced onion to make a bed for the stuffed tomatoes.
- Spoon the saucy meat and rice mixture into the empty tomato shells.
- Cover the stuffed tomatoes with the reserved tops.
- From one of the corners of your baking dish, carefully pour about ¾ cup of water.
- Add a little pinch of salt and a generous drizzle of extra virgin olive oil on top.
- Cover the baking dish with foil and bake in heated oven for 45 minutes.
- Uncover let cook for more 1 hour.

- When ready, serve and enjoy.

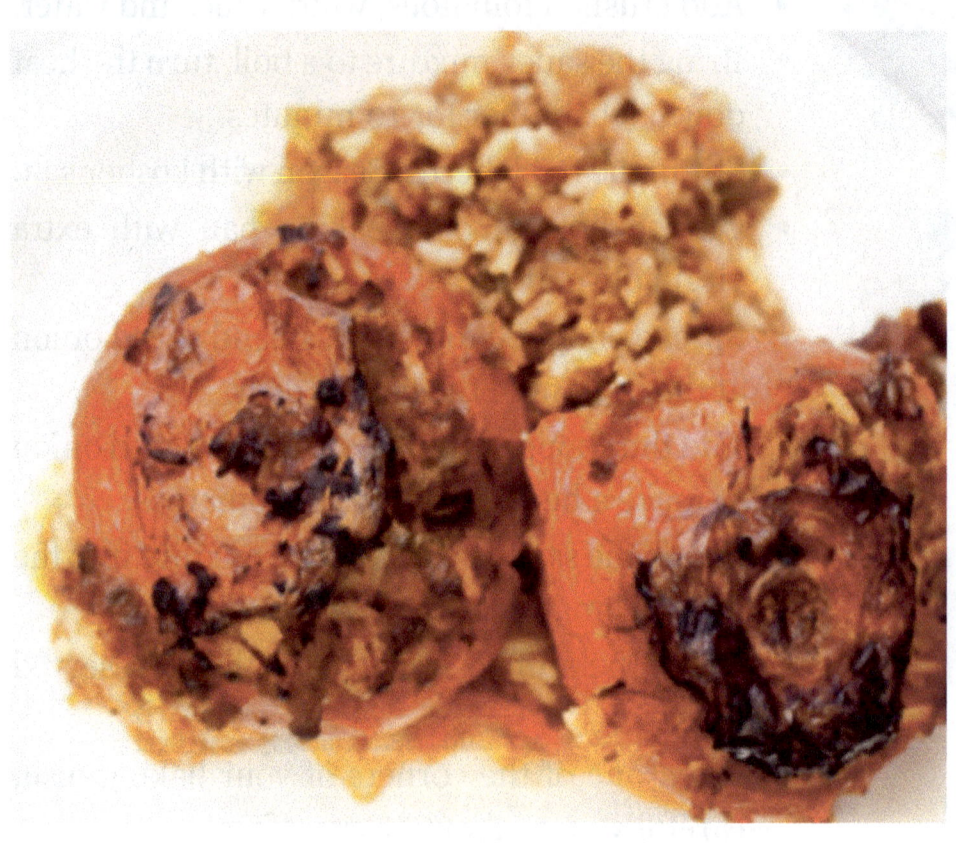

Carpers chicken

Although Mediterranean Sea diet focuses on fruits and vegetables, this carpers chicken is accompanied by rich vegetables.

Ingredients

- 1 lb. of boneless skinless chicken breasts
- 8 Fresh basil leaves
- Balsamic glaze or balsamic reduction
- Black pepper
- Extra virgin olive oil
- Kosher salt
- 4 slices low-sodium fresh mozzarella cheese
- Basil pesto
- 4 thick slices of ripe tomatoes

Directions

- Pat chicken dry and season with salt and pepper.
- Heat an indoor griddle then, drizzle with bit of extra virgin olive oil to coat bottom of pan.
- Place in the chicken let cook for 5 minutes on each side.
- At the last couple minutes of cooking, top each piece of chicken with a bit of the basil pesto, then add mozzarella slice on top.
- Remove from heat source.

- Add fresh basil leaves and tomato slices on top.
- Sprinkle with fresh basil ribbons.
- Serve and enjoy.

Mediterranean potato hash with asparagus, chickpeas and poached eggs

This is a colorful Mediterranean breakfast topped with chickpeas and poached eggs.

Ingredients

- ½ cup of crumbled feta
- 2 garlic cloves, chopped
- 2 russet potatoes, diced
- Salt and pepper
- 1 cup of chopped fresh parsley,
- 1 cup of canned chickpeas, drained and rinsed
- 1 small red onion, finely chopped
- 1 teaspoon of coriander
- 1 lb.. baby asparagus, hard ends removed, chopped into ¼ inch pieces
- Extra virgin olive oil
- 1 ½ tsp ground allspice
- 1 teaspoon of Za'atar
- 2 Roma tomatoes, chopped
- 1 teaspoon of dried oregano
- 1 small yellow onion, chopped
- Pinch sugar
- 4 eggs
- 1 teaspoon of sweet paprika
- Water

- 1 teaspoon of White Vinegar

Directions
- Heat olive oil in a large cast-iron skillet.
- Add the chopped onions, garlic and potatoes with the heat turned low.
- Season with salt and pepper let cook for 7 minutes, stirring frequently until the potatoes are tender.
- Add the chickpeas together with asparagus, a dash more salt and pepper and the spices. Stir to combine.
- Continue to cook for 7 minutes.
- Lower heat to keep the potato hash warm, stir regularly.
- Boil water to a steady simmer then add 1 teaspoon of vinegar.
- Break the eggs into a bowl.
- Stir the simmering water gently and carefully slide the eggs in let cook for 3 minutes.
- Season with salt and pepper.
- Remove the potato hash from the heat and add the chopped red onions, tomatoes, feta and parsley.
- Top with the poached eggs.
- Serve and enjoy.

Fried eggplant recipe with green peppers and tomatoes

Vegan, vegetarian alike, this recipe is a perfect option for vegans and vegetarians in love with awesome Mediterranean Sea diet.

Ingredients

- 2 large green bell peppers washed, dried, sliced
- 5 garlic cloves Roughly chopped
- 2 teaspoon of sumac
- ½ cup of fresh mint
- 2 teaspoon of white vinegar
- 6 large slicing tomato washed, dried, sliced in rounds
- ½ cup of healthy cooking oil
- 1 large eggplant washed, dried, sliced in rounds
- kosher salt
- ¼ cup of walnut hearts

Directions

- Spread eggplant slices on paper towels and sprinkle generously with kosher salt.

- Let sit for 30 minutes to sweat out any bitterness. Pat dry.
- Heat oil on medium-high heat let shimmer without smoke.
- Fry the green peppers, skin side down, until tender.
- Drain any excess oil, then sprinkle with a little salt and sumac.
- In the same frying pan, fry the eggplant flip over to balance the fry.
- Sprinkle with sumac.
- Then, fry the tomatoes for 2 minutes, add the garlic, let cook for 5 minutes, tossing gently.
- Lower the heat to add 2 tablespoons of vinegar, salt, and pinch of sumac.
- Turn heat off when tomatoes are releasing juices and turning bright orange.
- Layer a bit of the eggplant at the bottom, then add green peppers, then the saucy tomatoes on top.
- Repeat this step until the veggies are all on the platter.
- Garnish with fresh mint and walnut hearts.
- Serve and enjoy with Lebanese rice.

Crunchy roasted chickpeas

This is a quickie Mediterranean diet snack. It requires few ingredients especially salt and olive oil for the roast.

Ingredients
- Kosher salt
- 2 15 ounces cans of chickpeas, drained and rinsed
- Extra virgin olive oil
- Seasoning of your choice

Directions
- Drain and pat dry chickpeas.
- Heat your oven to 400°F.
- Spread the chickpeas well on a bare baking sheet.
- Drizzle with extra virgin olive oil and season with kosher salt. Toss.
- Roast in heated oven for 35 minutes, shaking the pan every 10 minutes.
- When chickpeas turn a deeper golden brown and the exterior is nice and crispy, they are ready.
- Season roasted chickpeas.
- Serve and enjoy.

Mediterranean style okra recipe

So far, this is the most amazing recipe among the Mediterranean Sea diet. Combining okra with onions and garlic with hot peppers, lime juice is remarkably perfect for a Mediterranean meal.

Ingredients

- Juice of ½ lime
- 1 small onion chopped
- 1 tomato sliced into rounds
- 4 garlic cloves minced
- ½ cup of water
- 1 lb.. frozen or fresh cut of okra sliced into rounds
- Salt and pepper
- 1 teaspoon of ground allspice
- ½ teaspoon of coriander
- 2 small green chills
- ½ teaspoon of paprika
- Extra virgin olive oil
- 1 ½ cup of crushed tomatoes

Directions

- Begin by heating olive oil in a large skillet over medium-high until shimmering without smoke.

- Lower the heat, add the onions together with the garlic and chopped jalapeno peppers.
- Let cook for 5 minutes stir frequently.
- Add the okra and sauté for 7 minutes over medium-high heat.
- Season with kosher salt, black pepper and spices. Toss.
- Add the crushed tomatoes and water. Stir to combine.
- Add the tomato slices on top and boil.
- Lower the heat, cover most of the way let okra simmer for 20 – 25 minutes.
- Uncover and add juice of ½ lime accordingly.
- Remove from heat and serve over rice.
- Enjoy.

Mediterranean salmon and vegetable quinoa

This Mediterranean salmon vegetable recipe cannot be underestimated in regards to its protein content. It is fully packed with healthy protein from vegetables and roasted spices with salmon fillets.

Ingredients

- ¾ cup of English cucumbers, diced, seeded
- ½ teaspoon of kosher salt
- ¼ cup of red onion, finely diced
- zest of one lemon
- ½ teaspoon of kosher salt
- 1 cup of quinoa, uncooked
- ¼ teaspoon of black pepper
- 8 lemon wedges
- 1 teaspoon of cumin
- 4 basil leaves, thinly sliced
- 1 cup of cherry tomatoes, sliced in half
- ½ teaspoon of paprika
- 20 ounces of salmon fillets
- ¼ cup of parsley, chopped fresh

Directions

- Boil 1 cup of quinoa, water and salt in a medium saucepan.

- Cook at reduced heat for 20 minutes as instructed on the package till fluffy.
- Turn off the heat allow it to settle for 5 minutes covered.
- Mix in the tomatoes, cucumbers, basil, onions, and lemon zest.
- In another separate small bowl, combine cumin, salt, pepper, and paprika.
- Line a sheet pan with a foil, grease with olive oil.
- Move the salmon fillets to the pan. Make sure to coat evenly on each surface with spice mixture.
- Place the lemon wedges at the edges of the pan.
- Broil on high heat for 8 – 10 minutes with the rack placed in the lower third of the oven till salmon is ready.
- Sprinkle with parsley.
- Serve and enjoy with roasted lemon wedges and vegetable quinoa.

Vegan tofu tikka masala

Tons of rich flavors feature in this Mediterranean vegan dish. This recipe using sesame oil and coconut milk in the place of butter making it a healthier option for your meal.

Ingredients
- ½ large head of cauliflower
- 1 ¼ teaspoon of Sea Salt
- Salt and pepper to taste
- ½ cup of red onion finely diced
- ½ cup full fat coconut milk
- ¼ cup of fresh ginger finely grated
- 1 ½ teaspoon of paprika
- 12 ounces extra firm tofu
- 1/8 teaspoon of nutmeg
- ¼ teaspoon of cayenne pepper
- 1 ½ teaspoon of ground cumin
- 4 cloves garlic minced
- 2 14 ounce cans of diced tomatoes
- ½ teaspoon of turmeric
- cilantro to garnish
- 3 teaspoon of sesame oil

Directions
- Begin by preparing your tofu by draining excess liquid.

- Wrap well within paper towels with a heavy material put on it for at least 10 minutes.
- In a skillet over medium temperature, add sesame oil followed by cubed tofu pieces.
- Season briefly with sea salt and pepper flip to let brown.
- Remove from pan.
- Add chopped garlic, onions, and grated ginger in the sesame oil balance.
- Sauté for 5 minutes until onions are translucent.
- Add all spices to the pan, including onion and ginger mixture.
- Pulse diced tomatoes in a blender, process until somewhat smooth.
- Transfer tomatoes into the pan, stir to combine.
- Add the tofu in, simmer for 10 minutes over low heat.
- Then add coconut milk, warm on low boil.
- Season with cayenne and sea salt.
- Place cauliflower in a food processor bowl.
- Process until broken into pieces.
- Add sesame oil and cauliflower over high heat.
- Sauté briefly for 3 minutes.
- Season with sea salt and pepper.

- Serve tofu tikka masala over cauliflower and enjoy with cilantro.

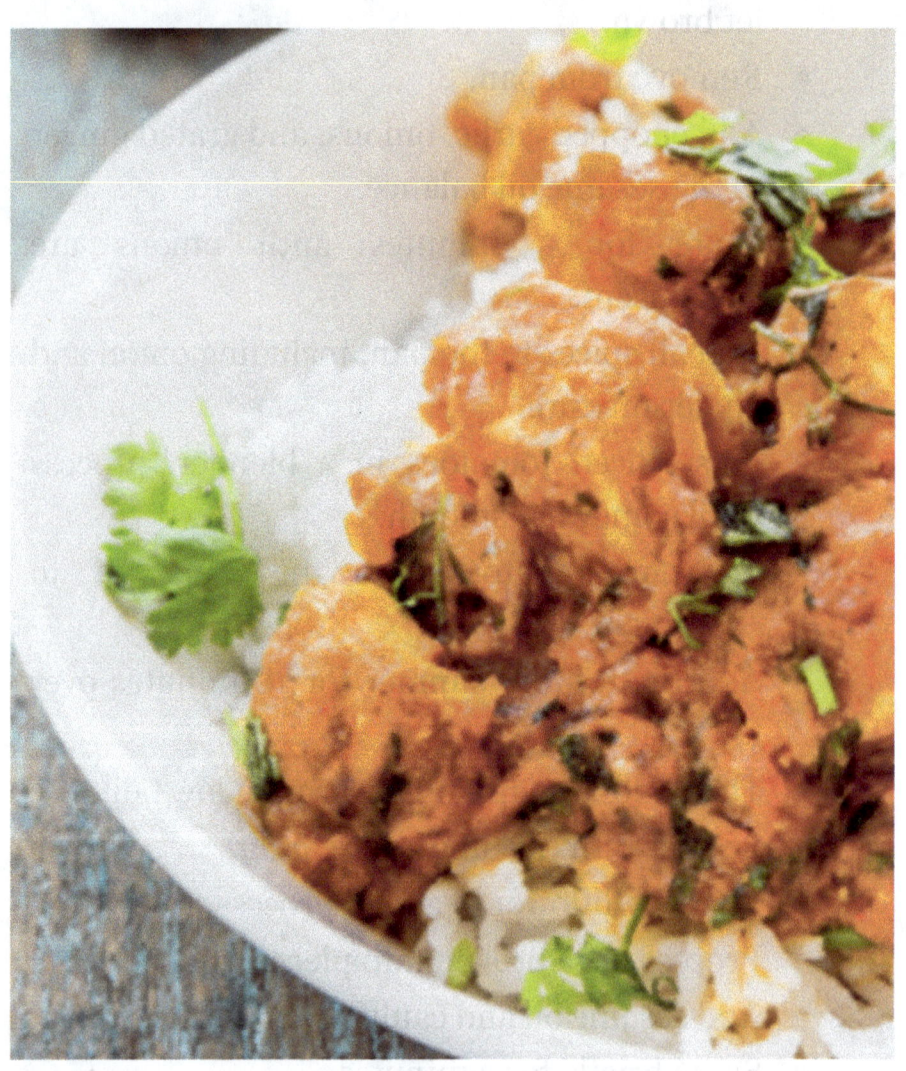

Mediterranean couscous

This couscous recipe is typically with nutritious flavors from herbs, zippy lemon, variety of veggies. As such, this is a versatile recipe for breakfast, lunch and dinner.

Ingredients

- ⅓ cup of extra virgin olive oil
- 2 garlic cloves, minced
- ½ English cucumber, finely chopped
- Salt and pepper
- [Private Reserve](#) extra virgin olive oil
- Water
- 2 cups of grape tomatoes, halved
- 3 oz. fresh baby mozzarella
- 15 oz. can of chickpeas, drained and rinsed
- 14 oz. can of artichoke hearts
- 1 teaspoon of dill weed
- ⅓ cup of finely chopped red onions
- 1 large lemon juice
- 2 cups of Pearl Couscous
- ½ cup of pitted Kalamata olives
- 15-20 fresh basil leaves, roughly chopped

Directions

- Put vinaigrette ingredients in a bowl. Whisk all to combine.

- In a medium-sized pot, heat 2 tablespoons of olive oil.
- Let couscous Sauté in the olive oil shortly to turn golden brown.
- Next, add 3 cups of boiling water continue to cook as per package instruction.
- Drain and keep for later.
- In a separate large mixing dish, combine all ingredients except basil and mozzarella.
- Add couscous with the basil mix.
- Whisk the lemon-dill vinaigrette. Add to couscous salad.
- Mix to combine.
- Test and season accordingly.
- Blend in the mozzarella cheese and finally garnish with basil.
- Serve and enjoy.

Stuffed peppers

The recipe derives its taste from rich meat packed with flavors and herbs as well as chickpeas. It a gluten free vegetarian dish for dinner and lunch or breakfast.

Ingredients
- 1 can of cannellini beans, drained and rinsed
- 4 cloves garlic, minced
- ½ cup of Feta cheese
- 5 cups of low-sodium vegetable broth
- 1 can of diced tomatoes
- 1 cup of carrots diced
- 1 cup of faro, rinsed
- 1 tablespoons of fresh lemon juice
- 1 cup of chopped celery
- 1 teaspoon of dried oregano
- 1 bay leaf
- 1 cup of chopped yellow onion
- Salt
- 2 tablespoon of olive oil
- ½ cup of packed parsley sprigs
- 4 cups of packed chopped kale

Directions
- Begin by heating oil over medium-high heat in a large pot.

- Next, add carrots, onion and celery, let Sauté for 3 minutes.
- Add garlic Sauté briefly.
- Stir in faro, vegetable broth, oregano, tomatoes, bay leaf, season with salt accordingly.
- Add parsley to the soup, let boil over low heat.
- Cover let simmer for 19 – 21 minutes.
- Remove parsley to stir in kale and kale, let cook for 13 – 15 minutes.
- Add cannellini beans, heat for 1 minute.
- Discard bay leaf and stir in lemon juice with extra vegetable broth.
- Serve warm and enjoy topped with feta cheese.

Easy Falafel meal

Ingredients
- Lemon
- ¼ teaspoon of Garlic Powder
- pinch each salt & pepper
- ½ cup of white onion
- ¼ cup of oat flour
- 2 tablespoons of tahini
- 3-4 tablespoons of avocado oil
- 4 cup of lettuce
- 2 tomatoes diced
- 1.5 teaspoon cumin
- 1/3 cup of chopped fresh parsley
- 1 Cucumber diced
- 1-15 ounce can chickpeas drained and rinsed
- 1 red onion sliced thin

Directions
- Add chickpeas, parsley, garlic powder, onions, tahini, cumin, and pepper to a blender, pulse to combined.
- Add oat flour pulse again.
- Then over high temperature, heat a large skillet with avocado oil.
- Scoop out falafel mixture, form into patties.

- Add falafel patties after the pan has heat up, let cook for 5 minutes.
- Repeat for all falafel patties until they turn golden brown.
- Divide lettuce, cucumber, tomato, and red onion in 4 dishes.
- Add falafel on top.
- Serve and enjoy with tahini or lemon.

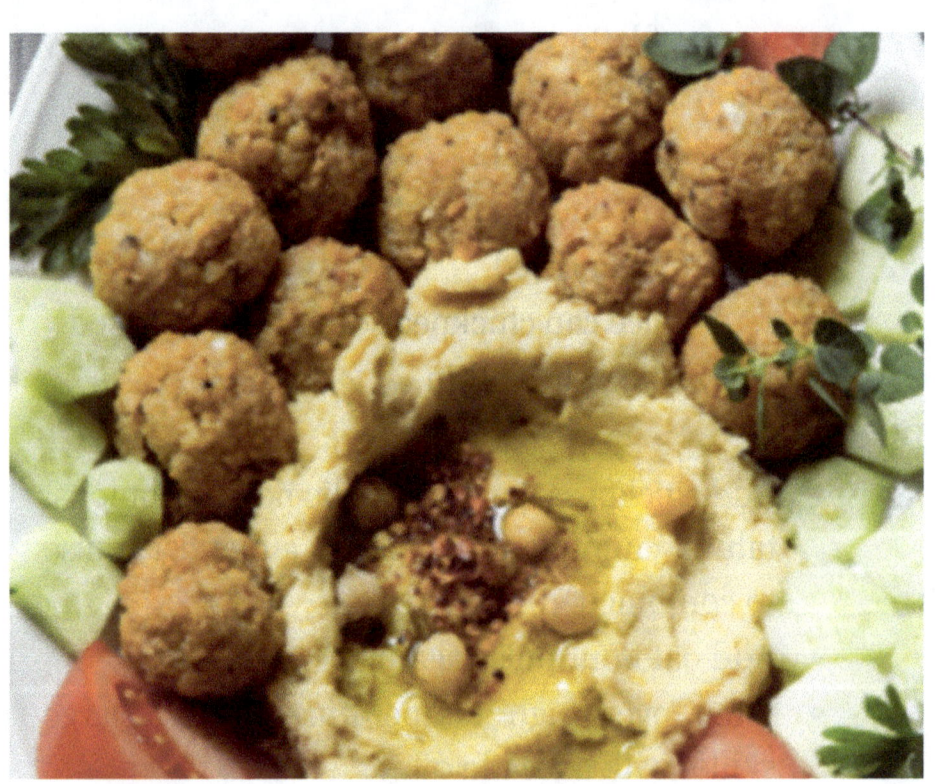

Pan seared salmon

To sear salmon, you need warm variety of spices which can be topped with a salsa fresca a Mediterranean style. Furthermore, the other ingredients used to make this recipe are quite simple especially garlic, pepper, cumin and coriander.

Ingredients

Pan Seared Salmon

- 1 teaspoon paprika
- ½ teaspoon ground cumin
- 1 teaspoon grated lemon zest
- ½ teaspoon ground coriander
- ¼ teaspoon salt
- ½ teaspoon granulated onion
- ¼ teaspoon black pepper
- Olive or avocado oil
- 4 salmon fillets skinned
- Pinch cayenne pepper
- 1 teaspoon granulated garlic

Mediterranean Salsa Fresca

- ¼ yellow bell pepper, finely diced
- 2 tablespoons finely diced red onion
- Black pepper
- 1 teaspoon chopped fresh dill
- 1 teaspoon chopped flat-leaf parsley

- Salt
- 2 tablespoons pitted Kalamata olives, diced
- 1 cup small cherry or sugar tomatoes, quartered
- ½ teaspoon grated lemon zest
- 1 small Persian cucumber, finely diced
- 1 teaspoon lemon juice

Toasted Couscous
- 1 tablespoon olive oil
- 1 cup couscous
- 1 tablespoon chopped parsley
- 1 clove garlic, pressed through garlic press
- 1 ¼ cup water
- Couple pinches of salt

Directions
- Firstly, Place the salmon fillets onto in a large bowl
- Drizzle 2 tablespoon of oil, sprinkle with paprika, cumin, garlic, onion, salt, coriander, pepper, cayenne and lemon zest, and toss.
- Let marinate for not less than 1 hour.
- As you wait for the salmon, combine all ingredients mix to combine. Ensure to keep refrigerated when covered.
- Again put another medium saucepan to heat over medium temperature.

- Add in the couscous and toast for 1 minute. Remove and keep for later.
- In the same pan, add water with salt, olive oil, and garlic. Stir to combine.
- Simmer thoroughly.
- Pour in couscous, stir.
- Turn off heat, leave covered for 4 – 7 minutes to soften.
- Add the chopped parsley, make sure it stays warm.
- Put a large skillet to heat spread with oil.
- Add in salmon fillets, let them sear on every side for 4 – 5 minutes. Repeat step for the other side.
- Top seared salmon with Mediterranean Salsa Fresca.
- Serve and enjoy.

One pan baked cod and vegetables

Ingredients
- 3 - 4 tablespoon of oil of choice
- 1 pound of Atlantic cod divided into 4 pieces
- 2 cups of purple potatoes diced
- 2 cups of Cherry Tomatoes

Directions
- Begin by preheating your oven to 400°F.
- Toss diced potatoes with in oil
- Roast for 15 minutes in the preheated oven.
- Remove pan from the oven to add in tomatoes and cod.
- Drizzle with remaining oil and season accordingly.
- Take back to the oven let it bake for more 10 – 12 minutes
- Serve and enjoy.

Quinoa bowls with roasted pepper

This recipe blends variety of veggies and herbs with quinoa, cheese, pepperoncini and olives for a delicious meal that you will not forget in ages.

Ingredients
- 1 clove garlic
- Hummus
- ½ teaspoon salt
- Sliced red onion
- ½ cup olive oil
- Pepper
- Kalamata olives
- Cooked quinoa
- Spinach, kale, or cucumber
- Juice of one lemon
- Feta cheese
- Pepperoncini
- ½ cup almonds
- Fresh basil or parsley
- 1 16 ounce of jar roasted red peppers, drained

Directions
- Combine red pepper, garlic, salt, lemon juice, olive oil, and almonds in a food processor.
- Blend until smooth.

- Next cook the quinoa according to package Directions.
- Build a Mediterranean Quinoa Bowl.
- Serve and enjoy.

Sweet potato wedges with tahini

This fried potato wedges make a perfect healthy snack. You can choose to dip in a sauce of your choice. The spices used here are almost addictive keeping you hooked onto eating every time and every time.

Ingredients

- ½ teaspoon of smoked paprika
- ½ teaspoon of olive oil
- 2 medium sweet potatoes
- ½ teaspoon of Chili Powder
- Salt and pepper
- ½ teaspoon of cumin
- 2 teaspoon of runny tahini

Directions

- Preheat your oven to 400°F.
- Align a baking sheet with parchment paper inside.
- Cut sweet potatoes in half, then each into 4 – 6 wedges.
- Organize the wedges on the baking sheet.
- Drizzle with the olive oil.
- Then sprinkle with salt, chili powder, pepper, and smoke paprika.
- Roast in the oven until brown and crispy in 35 – 40 minutes.

- Remove from the oven, let cool briefly.
- Serve and enjoy with runny tahini.

Armenia losh kebab

Unlike the common kebabs one can find in any restaurant around the corner, the Armenia losh kebabs are rare to find. You be lucky to find one in a restaurant menu. So use this recipe to make for yourself this delicious kebab.

Directions

- 1 cup of fresh parsley, chopped
- 1 lb. of ground beef
- ¾ cup of chopped parsley
- ½ white onion, chopped
- 1 lb. of ground lamb
- 1 white onion, chopped
- 1 tablespoon of cumin
- Juice of ¼ lemon
- 1 tablespoon of extra virgin olive oil
- 1 egg
- ¼ cup of tomato sauce
- Salt and pepper

Directions

- In a bowl, combine ground beef together with the lamb, onion, egg, parsley, lemon, cumin, olive oil, tomato sauce, salt and pepper.
- Form into burger patties keep for later.
- Next, heat your grill to medium high heat.

- Grill the burgers, make sure to flip once. Put aside to rest.
- Chop the remaining onion and parsley place in a bowl and let combine.
- Put your burger in a pita wrap.
- Use the parsley and onion mixture for topping. Wrap.
- Enjoy.

Eggplant, lentils and pepper cooked in olive oil

This is another 100 percent vegetarian recipe for a perfect Mediterranean Sea diet packed with bright flavors to tease your taste buds.

Ingredients

- 2 medium eggplants
- 1 red bell pepper, cut in half and thinly sliced
- Freshly ground black pepper
- 2 medium onions, halved and thinly sliced
- 14 ounces can of diced tomatoes
- 7 tablespoons of extra virgin olive oil
- 6 ounces of green lentils, rinsed
- 1 cup of water
- 1 teaspoon of salt
- 2 teaspoons of dried mint
- 4 cloves of garlic, crushed and finely chopped
- 1 teaspoon of granulated sugar

Directions

- Place in a boiling water to simmer when covered for 15 minutes.
- Drain out any excess water. Keep aside for later.
- Peel the eggplant and cut in half lengthwise.

- Spread on a wide tray then sprinkle with salt keep for 15 minutes.
- Drain excess water in the eggplants using a pepper towel.
- Next, heat olive oil 3 teaspoons in a pan, Sauté briefly for 2 minutes.
- In a large bowl, combine half way cooked lentils with the onion, bell peppers, garlic, tomatoes, dried mint, salt, olive oil, and sugar.
- Season with black pepper to taste.
- In another pan, place a layer of eggplant slices.
- Spread evenly with half of the vegetable mixture.
- Top with the remaining.
- Add water let cook for 36 minutes while covered over low heat.
- Serve and enjoy with crusty breads.

Potato omelet

Ingredients

- 10 eggs
- 1 onion, sliced in rounds, same thickness as potatoes
- ¾ cup extra virgin olive oil
- Salt and pepper
- 4 potatoes, peeled and sliced into rounds

Directions

- Add olive oil in a skillet frying pan.
- Add sliced potatoes when the oil is hot enough.
- Turn occasionally until it changes color to brown.
- Add onions to the potatoes after 10 minutes of frying.
- Sprinkle with salt and pepper.
- Fry further until tender all way through.
- In another large separate bowl, add the eggs, whisk until smooth.
- Turn on broiler in oven.
- Transfer content to a bowl.
- Let cool.
- Add oil in the skillet to covered every part in the skillet.

- Add potato mixture to egg mixture in bowl blend.
- Add salt and ground black pepper to the mixture.
- Place in the skillet.
- Cook until eggs start to set on bottom over medium heat.
- Continue to cook in the top rack of oven till eggs are set
- Remove, serve and enjoy.

Eggs poached in spicy tomato sauce, the Moroccan style

Ingredients
- 1 teaspoon of cumin
- 2 tablespoons of extra virgin olive oil
- Salt and pepper
- 3 cloves garlic, chopped
- 4 – 6 eggs
- 4 tomatoes of chopped
- 1 red pepper, chopped
- 1 onion, chopped
- ¼ cup fresh oregano, chopped
- 1 jalapeno of pepper, chopped
- 1 teaspoon of smoked paprika

Directions
- Heat oil in a medium skillet.
- Sauté onion together with the garlic for 1 minute.
- Next, add the red pepper. Sauté for 2 minutes.
- Add jalapeno pepper and also sauté for 30 seconds max.
- Add cumin, tomatoes, and smoked paprika to simmer for 15 – 20 minutes.
- Season with salt and pepper.
- Gently stir in oregano.

- Finally, break the eggs pour to mixture.
- Continue to simmer until the egg begins to set.
- Add more salt and pepper, to taste.
- Serve and enjoy.

Briam baked vegetables in olive oil

Ingredients
- 1 cup feta, crumbled
- 3-4 small zucchini, ends cut off and cut into pieces
- 2 onions, cut in half
- 1 teaspoon salt
- 1 red pepper, cut into pieces
- 1 orange pepper, cut into large pieces
- 4 small or 2 large potatoes, peeled cut into pieces
- 2 tomatoes, chopped
- 1 bunch dill, chopped
- 2 small or 1 large eggplant, cut into large strips
- ½ cup extra virgin olive oil

Directions
- Preheat oven to 400°F.
- In a large baking dish, mix all ingredients apart from feta.
- Cover with a lid, let bake for 1 hour as your keep stirring occasionally.
- Stir in feta cheese when off the heat.
- Serve immediately.
- And enjoy.

Eggplant parmesan with prosciutto

It is a lot of fun to prepare this recipe traditional style with no bread crumbs with lettuce, tomatoes, and cucumber for a healthy Mediterranean meal in about 1 hour.

Ingredients

- 2 medium sized eggplants
- Olive oil
- Salt and pepper
- Butter
- 1 Cup of tomato sauce
- 6 ounces of thinly sliced, raw Parma Ham
- 1 Cup of grated Parmesan cheese

Directions

- Begin by simmering the tomato sauce over low heat.
- Whereas, prepare the eggplant, cut into rounds.
- Sprinkle with salt, put in a colander for 20 minutes, wash, pat dry.
- Heat olive oil in a saucepan and place the eggplant slices to fry on every slide until brown.
- Using a paper towel, dry off.
- Place a layer of eggplant slices at the bottom of a buttered baking bowl.

- Cover with ham, pepper, tomato sauce, and Parmesan cheese.
- Repeat until ingredients are used up.
- Bake in a slow oven at 325°F after dotting with butter on the surface for 1 hour.
- Serve and enjoy when still hot.

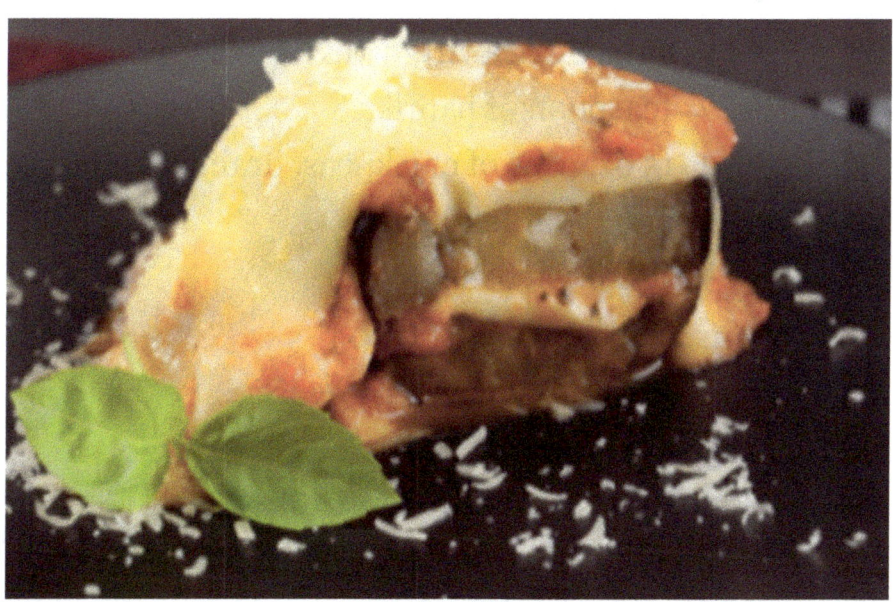

Lebanese hummus

This is another traditional recipe of the Mediterranean Sea diet prepared with garlic, extra virgin olive oil, lemon juice and paprika for a tasty meal to remember.

Ingredients

- 2 garlic cloves, crushed
- pine nuts for garnish
- 3 tablespoon of cold water
- 1/3 cup of freshly squeezed lemon juice
- ¼ cup of extra virgin olive oil
- ¼ teaspoon of paprika
- 2 -15 oz. cans of chickpeas, drained and rinsed
- ¼ cup of tahini paste
- ½ teaspoon of salt

Directions

- Begin by chopping the garlic and place in a food processor.
- Add the rest of the remaining ingredients.
- Blend until desired consistency.
- Serve and enjoy when smooth.

Grilled swordfish with lemon parsley topping

The lemon used in preparing this dish gives it all the flavor you are seeking for. It is quite easy to make in 10 minutes.

Ingredients
- Salt and pepper
- ½ cup of chopped parsley
- ½ cup of chopped onions
- ½ cup of extra virgin olive oil
- 1 ½ pounds of swordfish steaks
- ½ cup of fresh lemon juice

Directions
- Wash and pat dry the swordfish.
- combine onions, olive oil, lemon juice, parsley, salt and pepper in a small bowl.
- Place on the until firm to the touch in 5 minutes.
- Remove, then top with lemon parsley mixture.
- Serve and enjoy.

Orange lemon potatoes

This lemon potatoes recipe uses garlic, oregano, thyme, and lemon juice among others for a flavorful meal.

Ingredients
- Salt and pepper, to taste
- ½ cup of freshly squeezed lemon juice
- 1 cup of water
- 1 clove garlic, minced
- 2 tablespoons of mustard
- 1 ½ pounds of potatoes, peeled cut to quarters
- ½ teaspoon of dried oregano
- 1 cup of freshly squeezed orange juice
- ¾ cup of extra virgin olive oil
- ½ teaspoon of dried thyme

Directions
- Preheat your oven to 350°F.
- Add every ingredient to a baking pan.
- Mix with hands.
- Salt and pepper accordingly.
- Bake until potatoes are golden brown.
- Serve and enjoy.

Chickpea patties with sesame, cilantro and parsley

Ingredients
- 1 leek, cut into small chunks
- Extra virgin olive oil
- 1 bunch parsley, stems removed
- 1 onion cut into quarters
- 1 tablespoon dry coriander powder
- 1 pound dried chickpeas, soaked overnight
- 6 cloves garlic
- ½ teaspoon cumin
- 1 bunch cilantro, stems removed
- Salt and pepper
- 1 tablespoon baking soda
- Sesame seeds

Directions
- Rinse and drain soaked chickpeas.
- Add garlic, parsley, leek, onion, and cilantro to a food processor.
- Process until onion and garlic are pulverized.
- To the food processor, add the chickpeas with baking soda, coriander powder, cumin, salt and pepper.
- Ensure not to over blend the mixture.

- Place mixture in a refrigerator for not less than an hour.
- Form flat patties out of the mixture.
- Roll in sesame seeds.
- Add extra virgin olive oil to a frying pan, let heat over medium temperature.
- Fry patties until brown on every side.
- Drain on paper towels.
- Serve immediately and enjoy.

Shrimp with feta and tomatoes

Ingredients

- Salt and pepper, to taste
- 1 red pepper, thinly sliced
- ½ pound of feta, cut into small cubes
- 1 large onion, sliced
- ¼ cup extra virgin olive oil
- 2 cloves garlic, minced
- 2 fresh tomatoes, cut into small cubes
- 1 pound of medium sized shrimp, shells removed and de-veined

Directions

- In a large heavy frying pan, sauté the onion together with the pepper, and garlic for 5 minutes in olive oil.
- Add the tomatoes let it simmer for 15 minutes.
- Add the shrimp and cook for 10 minutes over medium heat.
- Add the feta also let it simmer for 5 minutes or so.
- Salt and pepper.
- Serve and enjoy.

Seared scallops with lemon orzo

It is worth serving this impressive meal with green salad, garlic and white wine. The scallops are seared with orzo for a tastier meal.

Ingredients
- Cooking spray
- 1 ½ pounds of sea scallops
- ¼ teaspoon of black pepper
- 1 cup of uncooked orzo
- 2 teaspoons of olive oil
- 1 cup of fat-free, less-sodium chicken broth
- ½ cup of dry white wine
- ¼ teaspoon of salt
- ¼ teaspoon of dried thyme
- 2 tablespoons of fresh lemon juice
- ½ cup of chopped onion
- 2 tablespoons of chopped fresh chives

Directions
- Start by heating a medium saucepan over medium temperature coated with cooking spray.
- Add onion to pan and sauté for 3 minutes.
- Place in the pasta, wine, broth, and thyme let boil at reduced heat to simmer for 15 minutes to absorb all the liquid.

- Place in the chopped chives with the lemon juice.
- Heat oil in another large skillet over medium heat.
- Sprinkle scallops evenly with salt and pepper.
- Then add them to the pan let cook for 3 minutes until done.
- Serve and enjoy with the pasta mixture.

Pasta with sundried tomato pesto and feta cheese

This is a simplified pasta dish with vegetables especially dry tomatoes, almond, garlic and herbs mainly basil. It makes a perfect spiced meal with rich flavor consistence.

Ingredients
- ½ teaspoon of salt
- ¾ cup of oil-packed sun-dried tomato halves, drained
- ½ cup of crumbled feta cheese
- 2 tablespoons of shredded Parmesan cheese
- 1 tablespoon of bottled minced garlic
- ¼ cup of packed basil leaves
- 2 tablespoons of slivered almonds
- ¼ teaspoon of black pepper

Directions
- Begin by cooking pasta as per the package directions
- Drain any excess water. Remember to keep 1 cup of the cooking liquid.
- Return pasta to the cooking pan.
- Put tomatoes together with basil leaves, almond, parmesan cheese, garlic, and salt in a food processor as the pasta cooks.
- Process until all chopped.

- Combine tomato mixture with the pasta water.
- Stir and whisk.
- Then, add to pasta and toss.
- Sprinkle feta on top.
- Serve and enjoy.

Linguine with garlicky clams and peas

The linguine with garlicky clams and peas recipe is tossed with vegan green salad to spice the whole meal. It draws its flavorful aroma from the garlic and basil among other flavors.

Ingredients

- 2 tablespoons of chopped fresh basil
- 2 tablespoons of olive oil
- 3 cans of chopped clams, undrained
- ¼ cup of dry white wine
- 1 ½ teaspoons of bottled minced garlic
- ¼ teaspoon of crushed red pepper
- 1 package of fresh linguine
- 1 cup of frozen green peas
- 1 cup of organic vegetable broth
- ½ cup of shredded Parmesan cheese

Directions

- Cook pasta as per the package directions.
- Drain any excess water.
- Secondly, heat oil in a large skillet over medium-high heat.
- Add to garlic to sauté for 1 minute.
- Drain clams but keep at least 1 cup of the cooking water for later.

- Add reserved water to broth, wine, and pepper in the pan and boil.
- Lower heat to simmer for 5 minutes as you stir infrequently.
- Add clams with peas let cook for 2 minutes.
- Add pasta and toss.
- Sprinkle with cheese and basil.
- Serve and enjoy.

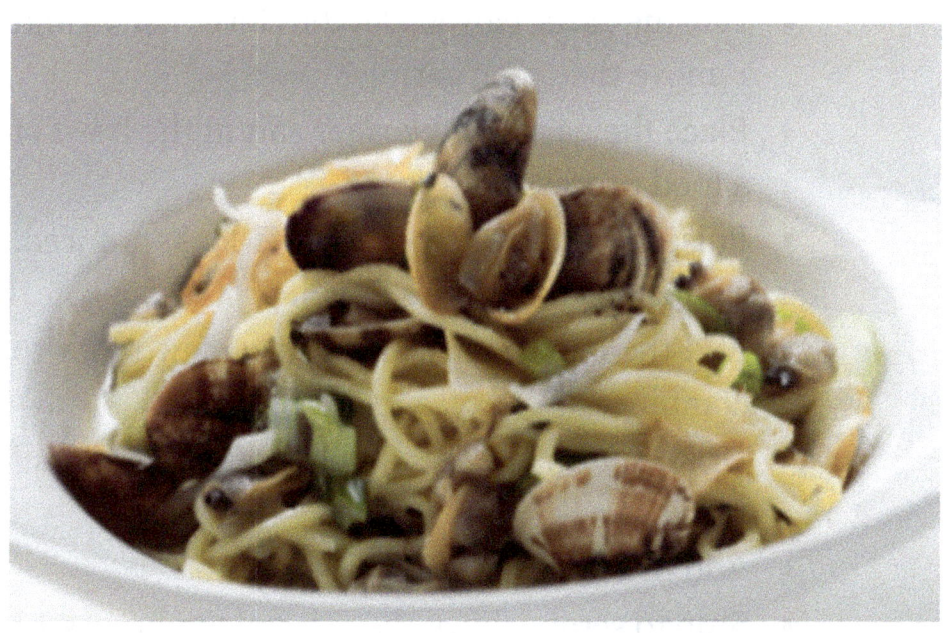

Toum garlic sauce

It is a smooth garlic sauce with garlic flavor throughout the sauce. It is versatile enough to spread and eat with anything whether shawarma, kofta, and falafel among others.

Ingredients

- 1 ¾ cups of grape seed oil or sunflower oil
- 1 teaspoon of kosher salt
- 6 tablespoon of ice water
- 1 head garlic
- 1 lemon juice

Directions

- Peel the garlic cloves. Cut the cloves in half and remove the green germ.
- Place the garlic and kosher salt in the bowl of a food processor.
- Pulse a briefly until the garlic looks minced, scrape down the sides as you process.
- Add the lemon juice and pulse a few times to combine.
- Drizzle with oil in as the processor is still running.
- Add in 1 tablespoon of the ice water.
- Stop to scrape down the sides of the processor bowl.

- Keep the processor running as you continue to slowly drizzle in the oil.
- Endeavor to add a tablespoon of the ice water after every ¼ cup of oil.
- Continue with this process until you have used up all the oil.
- Serve and enjoy.

Eggplant rollatini recipe

This recipe uses a tasty part-skim ricotta cheese filling with herbs parked in red sauce to tease you taste buds. It is a perfect Mediterranean Sea vegetarian diet.

Ingredients

- 2 tablespoons of basil pesto homemade
- Extra virgin olive oil
- 2 cups of Store-bought Marinara sauce
- 1 cup chopped fresh parsley leaves
- 3 tablespoons of grated Parmesan
- Salt
- 2 eggplants
- 2 eggs beaten
- 1 cup of part-skim ricotta cheese
- ½ cup of part-skim shredded Mozzarella

Directions

- Start by slicing the eggplants length-wise.
- Sprinkle eggplant slices with salt and keep aside on paper towel for 20 minutes.
- Pat dry. Rinse with water, then dry again.
- Heat your oven to 375°F.
- Brush a large baking sheet with extra virgin olive oil.
- Organize the eggplant slices in one layer on baking sheet.

- Brush the tops of the eggplant slices with more extra virgin olive oil.
- Bake in heated oven for 8 minutes until soft enough to fold.
- Remove from oven let cool shortly.
- In a bowl, add eggs together with the ricotta, grated Parmesan, Mozzarella, basil pesto, and fresh parsley. Mix to combined.
- Spread ¾ cup marinara sauce on the bottom of a baking dish.
- Scoop 2 tablespoons of the filling onto one end of each eggplant slice.
- Spread, starting from the short end, roll up eggplant slices tightly and arranged on prepared baking dish.
- Top eggplant rollatini with the remainder of the marinara sauce and a sprinkle of mozzarella.
- Bake in heated oven for 30 minutes until tender.
- Remove from oven let settle for 10 minutes.
- Serve and enjoy.

Vegetarian moussaka recipe

This recipe is also eggplant based entailing layers of roasted eggplants, zucchini, and potatoes with delicious Mediterranean tomato lentil soup.

Ingredients
- Salt
- 2 large zucchinis, sliced length-wise
- Extra virgin olive oil
- ½ teaspoon of nutmeg
- ⅔ cup of all-purpose flour
- Pinch of cinnamon
- 1 teaspoon of dry oregano
- 2 medium eggplants partially peeled and sliced length-wise
- ½ teaspoon of salt, more if you like
- ¼ teaspoon of ground nutmeg
- 4 cups of milk, warmed
- 2 large eggs
- 1 yellow onion, chopped
- 3 Russet potatoes, peeled and sliced lengthwise
- 2 garlic cloves, minced
- 1 ¼ cup of cooked black lentils
- 1 14-oz. can of crushed tomatoes

- ⅓ cup + 2 tablespoons of Greek extra virgin olive oil
- ½ cup of broth or water

Directions
- Heat your oven to 400°F.
- Spread eggplant slices on a large pan lined with paper towel and sprinkle with kosher salt, set aside for 20 to 30 minutes.
- Pat dry with paper towels
- In a large saucepan, heat olive oil over medium-high heat until shimmering without smoke.
- Stir in flour together with the salt and pepper let cook until golden.
- Gradually add the warmed milk, whisking continuously.
- Continue cooking, stirring occasionally, over medium heat for 7 minutes.
- Add nutmeg and in a small bowl, whisk a small amount of the hot béchamel mixture with the 2 eggs.
- Then return all to the pan with the balance of the béchamel mixture.
- Continue to whisk, then boil for 2 minutes.
- Taste and adjust salt and pepper.
- Remove from heat let allow to cool.

- In a large non-stick pan, heat 1 tablespoon of extra virgin olive oil over medium heat.
- Sauté onions together with the garlic briefly, tossing regularly.
- Stir in cooked black lentils together with the crushed tomatoes and broth.
- Season with a dash of kosher salt.
- Add oregano, nutmeg and a small pinch of ground cinnamon.
- Boil, then lower heat and cover part-way let simmer for 20 minutes.
- While lentil sauce is simmering, bake the vegetables. Arrange the potatoes, zucchini and eggplant slices on lightly oiled baking sheets. Brush with extra virgin olive oil. Bake in heated oven for 15 to 20 minutes just until tender.
- Pour bit of the lentil sauce on the bottom of the baking dish and spread.
- Layer the vegetables on top.
- Add the remainder of the lentil sauce and spread béchamel sauce on top, ensure it is smooth.
- Place moussaka casserole on the middle rack of your heated oven let bake for 45 minutes.

- Remove from heat, let sit for at 30 minutes before cutting.
- Serve and enjoy.

Honey mustard salmon recipe

This salmon is quite flaky covered or coated with sweet natural honey mustard sauce. It is flavored with garlic featuring other vegetables mainly paprika and cayenne.

Ingredients
- 2 ½ teaspoon of [Extra virgin olive oil](#)
- Lime wedges to serve
- ½ teaspoon of black pepper
- ½ teaspoon of cayenne
- Parsley garnish
- 4 tablespoons of whole grain mustard
- 2 tablespoons of [honey](#)
- 2 lb.. salmon fillet
- Kosher salt
- 4 garlic cloves minced
- 1 teaspoon of [smoked paprika](#)

Directions
- Firstly, heat your oven to 375°F.
- Pat dry the salmon fillet.
- Season with salt on both sides.
- In a small bowl, whisk together honey with whole grain mustard, minced garlic, extra virgin olive oil, smoked paprika, cayenne, and black pepper.
- Place the salmon on a lightly oiled sheet pan.

- Spread the honey mustard sauce evenly over the surface of the salmon.
- Cover with an aluminum foil bake for 20 minutes.
- Place under the broiler for 3 minutes uncovered.
- Place the seasoned salmon on a large, lightly oiled piece of aluminum foil.
- Spread the honey mustard sauce on top of the salmon.
- Fold both sides of the foil over the salmon and tightly close at the top.
- Place on a medium-high gas grill.
- Let cook for 10 – 12 minutes when covered.
- Open the top of the foil up so the fish is exposed.
- Cook for 3 more minutes.
- Remove from the heat source and squeeze a bit of fresh lime juice and garnish with parsley.
- Serve and enjoy.

Muhammara recipe/roasted red pepper dip

This is perfect substation or addition to the mezze table with baba ganoush and hummus served with pita bread or chips.

Ingredients
- 1 teaspoon of Aleppo pepper
- ¼ lb. shelled toasted walnuts
- ½ teaspoon of cayenne pepper
- ½ teaspoon of salt
- 1 garlic clove roughly chopped
- 2 ½ tablespoons of tomato paste
- ¾ cup of bread crumbs
- 2 tablespoons of molasses
- ½ teaspoon of sugar
- 4 tablespoons of extra virgin olive oil divided
- 2 red bell peppers
- 1 teaspoon of sumac

Directions
- Preheat your oven to 425°F.
- Brush the bell peppers with bit of olive oil.
- Place in a lightly oiled oven pan.
- Roast for 30 minutes turn over occasionally.
- Remove and place the peppers in a bowl.
- Cover with plastic wrap for a few minutes.

- When cool enough to handle, peel the peppers, remove the seeds and slice the peppers into small strips.
- In the bowl of a large food processor, combine the roasted red pepper strips together with 3 tablespoons of extra virgin olive oil, tomato paste, walnuts, bread crumbs, Aleppo pepper, pomegranate molasses, sugar, sumac, salt and cayenne.
- Blend into a smooth paste.
- Transfer to a serving bowl.
- Serve and top with a drizzle of extra virgin olive oil, and garnish with walnuts and fresh parsley, if desired.
- Enjoy with pita chips.

www.ingramcontent.com/pod-product-compliance
Lightning Source LLC
Chambersburg PA
CBHW070731030426
42336CB00013B/1937